HE AND I

HE AND I

JOURNEY FROM NEVERLAND
A STORY OF UNCONDITIONAL LOVE

Lesley Beck

Matador
Unit E2 Airfield Business Park,
Harrison Road, Market Harborough,
Leicestershire. LE16 7UL
Tel: 0116 2792299
Email: books@troubador.co.uk
Web: www.troubador.co.uk/matador
Twitter: @matadorbooks

ISBN 978 1803131 375

British Library Cataloguing in Publication Data.
A catalogue record for this book is available from the British Library.

Printed and bound in Great Britain by 4edge Limited
Typeset in 11pt Minion Pro by Troubador Publishing Ltd, Leicester, UK

Matador is an imprint of Troubador Publishing Ltd

This book is dedicated to my son, a gift

I, is Lesley Beck, a semi-retired counsellor and psychotherapist living amongst the same wonderful friends and neighbours for the last 35 years in West London. He, is her son, an accomplished drummer, a director of the Mango Mammals record label, a songwriter, a man of wit, skills and talent. He has Down's Syndrome, is on the autistic spectrum and lives in an assisted living community in East Sussex.

SLICK

It was supposed to be cranberry ice cubes and soft music
It's the beeps I remember
The rhythmic Morse code of machines
And then, absence of beeps
Punctured by the violence of voices, hands, feet, wheels
Lights a blur as we hurtle down the corridor
The urgency, the running, discordant noises, without rhythm
Metal on flesh, limbs, smells, the grasp, the pull, then
It's, it's like a bird in an oil slick
A moment caught in freeze frame
And silence, absolute terrifying silence, because
There should be a cry but
There is only silence
And then a sound, like slurping on a straw
And a tiny mewing
And we collectively breathe again

I am cold, shakingly, shockingly cold
Jabs, drips, steel
Where are you my little bird
Tarred and limp

Another freeze frame
Voices, faces peering, staring
Embarrassed, no or yes, yes embarrassed
But, for me, embarrassed for me because
I cannot now be admitted to the club
I have failed the criteria
There can be no welcoming fanfare for me

Later, much much later
People are called, contacts are made, details given
Minimal
The sex, the syndrome, the chosen name
To strained and false good cheer
But from you, an unexpected, chilling silence
And then
Oh dear me, oh dear dear me
Well I suppose I'll get used to it but
I do think you've chosen a very strange name
And I laughed, laughed aloud
For my oil slicked little bird
And his very strange name.

DOOR AJAR

Sometimes I glimpse who he so nearly was
Who he might have been, he
A kintsugi bowl
A piece of golden joinery
The one cannot exist without the other
Sometimes he walks hand in hand
With his shadow self
A sudden turn or tilt of the head
A smile full of wit or mischief
He looks me in the eye
Sharing a joke, an ingenious pun
Seated at his kit, he drums with skill and poise
Focused, alert, vibrant, assured and
Claiming his place in the scheme of things
Belonging
Sometimes his shadow self is hard to find
As if
On a trip from Neverland it has come adrift
Separated and held captive in a drawer
And I like Wendy
I try to sew this gossamer fabric
Delicate as cobwebs
Back where it belongs, uniting him
With his shadow self
But however gentle, the sewing can
Prick the skin

Cause pain fear anxiety
And he, he might abandon, fly away
Second star to the right
Straight on till morning
Without his shadow self
Into a perpetual childhood

A lost boy
Sometimes he glimpses his own shadow
Peering round a door, wondering
What is on the other side
In that other room
Is this where his shadow lives
A door that is never completely closed
But never completely opened either
Its contents as elusive as
Distant mist or seascape susurrations
He will peep and venture in with trepidation
A tentative visitor to a different world
One that entices but terrifies too
The join fragile, tenuous, so very delicate and
His beauty lies in this very flaw
So the door will stay ajar
But never fully open

IMPERFECT OFFERING

He fearful of food, it chokes him
A reflex taken for granted, he is having to learn
Little blue train a constant companion
Squeeze squeak cheekstroke swallow
A rhythmic pulse to each spoon tip bird like offering
Little blue train squeaks in approval

Kaleidoscope of colour, tapestry of texture
Overwhelms and terrifies
So each item a solo traveller
Isolated and lonely on its little plate
Bereft of a companion
Pasta no sauce on one
Courgette slice on two
Banana ring on three
Smoked salmon slither on four
Yoghurt spoonful on five
Nectarine segment on six
They must not touch
They must not meet
They must not mingle and assault the senses

I experiment
Such tentative visits, no fuss, no comment
Stealth practically invisible
Plate hopping is frowned upon
Screamed upon, hurled against the wall

Rejected for their lack of propriety
Each meal I attempt one small act of migration
Until we have
Four plates, then three, then two, then
One day just the one plate
Items not touching but one single plate
Little blue train squeaks with joy

Today there is no squeak, no train
Today no interfering voices tell me
He is attention seeking, being wilful
Must be forced to eat
Will never integrate
No today he and I and K and D
Slurp our 11 ingredient chow mein supper
Eaten with chop sticks
And he still chomping helps himself to seconds
He free of fear and loving food and
I give silent thanks to a little blue train

GAME CHANGER

Each week we gather in a circle
Cross legged on the floor
Our leader, guitar in hand
And hamper full of promise
A promise of sounds to come
Infants crawl, totter, shriek and run
He sits leaning against me
At times enchanted, at times alarmed
He does not crawl
Moves forward only, on his rump
Propelled by arms, looking surprised that he hovers not
Surprised too when he topples backwards
A visiting alien
Caught in a too powerful gravitational pull
Unable to change level or direction
And like the dalek defeated by stairs

We choose our instruments
There is never deviation in his choice
The little frog guiro has become his alone
His frustrated scream, alarm to others to stay away
Should another hand brush against what he has claimed
And other hands now clutch at
Bells, Rattles and Tambourines
Our leader begins to play
To sing the songs we have come to know so well

He leans against me I can feel his heartbeat
We stroke the rhythm along the little frog's ridges
He is at ease at one with the beat
We are at one with the rhythm
Our breath, our heartbeat exactly matched
A peaceful communion in this potential chaos
The tune, the rhythm, the beat, the breath
His causeway into this, our world
This beat, this rhythm is our Morse code
Our call and response, our language
A link, a bridge
He is not alone or silent
The rhymes and repetition a thread to remembrance
A handle and lever upon which to hang
This foreign language of words
Until words will have meaning, have purpose
And one day can and will be used
He will taste them, chew them
Watch them spill out

Sometimes as we sit in this, our circle
Amongst but not entirely part of
More apart
From this band of mothers and their chicks
A man comes with his son, a wheelchair user

They go up the gentle incline to sit
Looking out over the river, to simply be elsewhere
His son a young man, a journey already travelled
The shoes old, worn and familiar
I still have blisters and the pathway is unknown
I look at them and wonder
Wonder what exactly
It is too much

This day, session over
The mothers have gone
Gone to the park with their chicks
He is today reluctant to relinquish the frog
Our leader is patient
She understands, we talk, we wait
Until it flies into the hamper, it is home
He enjoys the now empty space
Doing the buttock shuffle
I have held him, arranged arms, legs, ready to crawl
Held between my knees and thighs
A miniature pony
Guiding first hand, then knee, as instructed
Oppositional movement defeats him

Oh to know then what I know now
The pain, the fear so much less
If I had but glimpsed
The skills, the grace that was to come
Instead each day a series of tasks
A ladder to climb

Today I see the man and his son
He is helping his son to take a drink
They do not speak
But love is there
Tangible as a shaft of light
Lifting the darkness

My back is turned
I fetch the pushchair
I am startled by a crow of delight
And turn
He is crawling up the three wide stairs
Is on the middle one
Facing upwards, moving upwards
Moving up the step, arms then legs
I am transfixed, amazed, struck dumb
To others such a little thing
To me a mountain climbed

I meet him at the top
And only when the man puts his hand upon my shoulder
"I know" he says
"I know how huge this is"
Only then do I realise my tears are falling
My top is wet with tears of hope
Tears of possibility, of gratitude
He is beaming his melon slice smile
He is so delighted to be there
And he knows that I know he knows
This is a game changer
He can explore that little bit more
He can go on an adventure

OCTOPUS

His peers have parties in pools, pavilions,
And pizza parlours
In pirate playgrounds and burger bars
On trampolines and bouncy castles
They leap, they twirl, they shriek and scream
And when invited we do accept
Wanting to be included
He hovers like a moth outside a window
Troubled by lights, the noise and bustle
Isolated in his exile of watching
At a distance
Observer of this other country
Confused by copious confounding customs

It is his sixth birthday
And we are home, not alone
Invites sent and accepted
His classmates sit all around
On sparkly silver blue tarpaulin
He too is seated in this circle
His eyes look huge, his mouth so round
The parcel goes from child to child
Unpeeling gently to cries of mirth
Thrilled by this game of long ago

Mr Bonkers has entertained
A gentle magic with his wand
Clown clothes but no clown make up
To frighten or to cause alarm
He is caring, kind, will come again
Calmed his act, spoke slow and clear
Never forgetting the birthday boy
Commotion in the ocean
Has been the theme
Napkins, plates, lunch boxes too
Star fish sandwiches and octopus cake
Tentacles cut into little slices

His party goes well
It is enjoyed
And he is at its epicentre
Now overwhelmed by people leaving
Retreats towards the kitchen door
And I distracted by departing guests
Leave him be for just a moment
A moment that has proved too lengthy
For here he sits centre table
Amidst a scene of much destruction
Amongst the detritus of his misdemeanour

A small green Buddha in this his kingdom of
Mangled tentacles and half chewed icing
Clumps of green held in each hand
Smeared in hair, on face, on limbs
Green froths, gurgles and pours from his mouth
A steady flow, a seaweed smile
He chortles with much glee
Delighted at this ending
To an almost perfect day
The octopus has been vanquished

HEROES

He chose one hero early
Seated before the TV screen
Plastic tambourine and wooden drum
Sticks poised to play along
Or newly minted from his bath
Modesty preserved by toy guitar
He stood transfixed by these
Great kings of rock
That rhythmic beat of ecstatic joy
To celebrate our being alive
And for some just having survived
Or the minor chord that weeps a flood
And gives voice to all our unshed tears
He laid full claim to chords and gods
And gazed upon Bruce Springsteen

Each week we drove the width of London
A full three hour round trip
For workshops, plays and story telling
With a theatre troupe of diverse grouping
And here he found another hero
Whose drumming skills were much sought after
For shows and gigs recordings too
And he would watch and swim a sea
Of pride and awe and downright envy

Seeing himself on his hero's kit
He made an art of his worship
Until one day in the theatre bar
He is rewarded with a gift
A weathered pair of sticks
Bearing the name of Simon Cooper

HERO NO MORE

You were his hero once
But now
In the slipstream of your detritus
Others are left to clear the pathways
From the scenes of your destruction
To juggle back the jigsaw pieces of a life
A life you leave fragmented in your wake

Your discordant tones harangue us
Your vain attempts to drown out truth or reason
Your worldview seen only through your shrunken prism
You hijack and distort the world's every season
You rob him of what is rightfully his
You move to justify your acts of treason

Not even warranting our rage
Only cold, hard, crystal hard contempt
At the foot stamping, the barking, the ranting and the railing
Your man-child goes rampaging through threads
That should be binding
You try to wipe the slate with a besmirched cloth
So your history is motheaten by distortion
And when shaken out, reveals its holes
The victim of an infestation

You seek entitlement without responsibility
You applaud yourself, others are silent
Can stay mute as you speak such volumes
And those who hear are not deceived
You only ask what can you take
Never what you might give

ALERT

London is on high terrorist alert
I am at work
He is on a holiday scheme outing
They are to go to a bowling alley
And will travel on the bus
He has freedom pass and packed lunch
His carers my emergency number
He knows them well and they know him
For the next five hours I will earn our living

My phone rings
He is stuck on the bus
Distressed, crying, refusing to move
Said bus is now at Terminal Five
At London's Heathrow Airport
London is on high terrorist alert
This is its final destination
And he is now in meltdown
Says the carer I know and trust
We are surrounded by armed police
The bus has been impounded
You need to come now and bring ID
Just tell them not to touch him
He will lash out if touched
I know, I know, she says
Come quick

Her paperwork shows she works for Mencap
I grab passports, DWP letter, water and
Bottle of rescue remedy, for me
I need to drive, cannot stop shaking
Keep calm, they will not shoot him or
Will they, I do not know
I drive like the proverbial
Bat out of hell
And hell is where I now reside
I have been instructed where to park
What route to take, registration number noted
I will be stopped and checked along the way
The airport is on high alert

My mouth dry, my back dripping
My hands still shaking, I am updating
The firearmed team as I drive
Infringing, trampling more laws
Than he has ever done, I can imagine
I can only imagine his fear
At all these guns and loud voices
I keep repeating, please just do not touch him
And they don't
My heart is thumping in my chest
This is so not the time to die

I arrive and they are kind
Which leaves me feeling humbled
But they are still armed, question me closely
Because someone somewhere might just think
To strap a suicide vest to a disabled young man
But not at this time and not this young man
I board the bus
He is huddled, fear bouncing off him
Hits me like a wave
Hi, this bus needs to be somewhere else, I say
Let's get off now and we can have lunch
So prosaic in its intent
A collective breath is held
Will he, won't he
He does
And we leave, disaster averted
And we do have lunch, the packed lunch
Sitting in the car, in a park
And I am still shaking

MOURNING

We are at the funeral of
She not my mother but the woman
Who held him that first Christmas
His first Christmas
When we but a few weeks out of hospital
After many weeks in hospital
And I so alarmed that I would fail
In this task of keeping him alive
The only nutrient he could tolerate was me
I stood between him and oblivion and
Was consumed with fermenting fear
And she, she understood how
Hard it was to let him out of my arms for a second
But there he nestled in hers
And now she was gone
And looking around me
So was he

We had tried to find ways
To make death somehow explicable
To make sense of such bone crunching loss
The weight of missing
The circle of life
That those we love live on in us
Our thoughts, our memories, part of us forever
Knowing them makes us who we are

And
We honour them by living well
By being the best we can
Where had he gone

Their dog had left this world before she did
And he scared of dogs had loved him
This creature, a psychiatrist in canine form
Had sensed his every mood, listened to his every word
Had kept his trust safe and secure
Age had lent him gravitas
He had no need to surprise or seek attention
Slow of movement, gentle of bark
He was an easy wise companion
They had held each other close
He was missed
And now lay buried in the meadow
And that was where we found him
Stroking the grass mound covering
Speaking of his latest loss

Sharing the day with his four legged friend
Unburdening himself of this, his further grief
Ensuring that his friend was not excluded
From this day of mourning
He had taken him a sausage

And we are undone,
Unravelled by this honest generous simplicity
We join him in this circle of love
Of the living and the dead
And mingle our tears
As we hold each other tight

BEST GIFT

I have been given
And have given
A great many gifts
But only rarely do you get to give
What someone really truly wants
Wants above all else
He wanted to play in a professional band
With those who did this for their living
To be amongst musicians
To be the drummer at a professional gig
To be the bee's knees, the cat's whiskers
To be it
And this could be my gift
My birthday, a significant one
So a party and a band
Friends and acquaintances wove a dream
Through acts of kindness big, small and massive
Turned dream to reality
They rehearsed, they played, he gave his all
He will, he does, can truly play
And he did, was whooped and cheered
He smiles, his smile of total joy
This man of substance, of talent and skill
Verily the best gift I have ever given
The best I have ever been given

AND THEN

All was ready
A night of toil, laughter and love
Behind us
Bales of hay, large cans raffia encircled
Bursting with flowers, leaves, petals abound
Glasses sparkle, tables are laid, plates stacked
It's time to dress
And he stands balanced on the apex of anxiety

I can't do this, he says
Breathe, I say, you can, you know you can
He hugs me tight, he so wants to, do this
Has thought of little else
Wants to look handsome but the shave is daunting
The sound, the feel of razor upon skin
He stands before me
Now clean of chin, so proud
In shirt, bootlace, jacket, trousers and shoes
It is time to find the groom

The groom who has grown a beard
Special for this day
You want to be handsome, he is told, like me
You need to shave and the groom does
Testament to his love

Anxiety rises he can do this
He will not let her down
And she is standing before him, so beautiful
She in her killer heels, his eyes just level with her chest
She takes his arm, gives it a squeeze and
He, he walks her down the aisle to greet
Her clean shaven groom
He beams, bathed in their love, so proud

A band is to play at the wedding feast
Delayed in their arrival
No time now to rehearse
With the guest they have been told
Will guest drum for three numbers
No worries the leader says, we know them well
And then he meets their guest drummer
This drummer now so anxious
He cannot even speak
But he sees the kit and smiles

The band too polite to comment, to question
And they are hired by bride and groom
Who are insistent that he will play
On this their most important day
He has not let go of his sticks
Holds them like a talisman
To ward off demons

The band just shrugs and prepares to, car crash
Invite him to the stage, adjust the kit
And begin to play and so does he
Country Roads, Brown Eyed Girl
The band's drummer stands at the side
Watching this usurper drum, he is astonished
His prejudices are undone
He catches the singer's eye
Fuck me, he can really play, he mouths
He can indeed, say I

DISCO

Disco night was his all time favourite
The certainty he would see his brown eyed girl
They both loved to dance, her height matched his exactly
Two peas in a pod

He pictured their life together
Like a lacemaker spinning fine threads of dreams
A future woven through the years ahead
A rich and vibrant tapestry

And for him the thought was as firm as the deed
His thoughts, so clear to him, how could she not
Think the same, want the same, dream the same
He believed and so it followed it must be
Ill at ease with squeezing feelings into words
And giving words to feelings
He let the music fill him up
Pulse through him like breath itself
He was the rhythm, the beat
He the heartbeat and she his heartsong
Dancing, holding his brown eyed girl
Grinning and glowing with the joy of living

Sometimes he would bring her flowers
She would raise them to her face
Thank you babe, love you, she always said
Sometimes they would go for a burger or to Pizza Express
Why would it ever change
It was all he wanted

For her words were feathers, fluttering things
Easily let go and forgotten
He tasted, ate words, savoured, relished them
Found with difficulty, they had weight
They were anchored
She was all light and frivolity
Flitting from flower to flower
He was all intensity and obsession
Tenacious as tar

This night she is standing with someone
Drink in hand
Laughing, looking up, up at this crusher of his dreams
And he, he is angry because this is not expected
Not what he has imagined, for him, for her
He cannot find the words
He cannot, will not share

He goes home to punch his fist into the wall
And he weeps, oh how he weeps, he sobs
He hurts so bad
He cries out
Why does it hurt so bad
When can we stop being broken up and be together again

He is hurting, his chest is hurting
He can feel his heart is breaking
A jigsaw of fragments he cannot put together
He clutches tight his broken heart
And his shattered dreams
And he weeps

HEARTSONG

He does not welcome touch
Unexpected or unsought
He will not often look you in the eye
Or even say hi
He may imply you intrude into his world
Leave you knocking gently to be admitted, unheeded
He could, hurl himself into a hug
At a time of his choosing
And you feel so honoured, so chosen, so blessed
He can smile into your eyes
And you will feel he has bestowed, entrusted you
Guardian of the finest joke in the whole world
And you are trusted to hold it and him safe
You have been honoured, you have been chosen
You are the one

But today is changed, parameters altered
For we are separated by fears and rules
Summoned to our sessions by a chirruping call
Accept, reject, leave message, chat
There is no touch, no hug, no wiping of tears of
Mirth or pain

To look into the camera's eye is today too much, extreme
I am greeted by side view of ear and
Fraction of smile that lights him up, hovers, a gift
Great news, he says and moves away to
Tell his tale, his grin a lurking shadow
I stare at his wall, hear his words, tune in to tone
And wait for his face to return or
Finger to finger
Separated by pane of glass
Is this how we navigate home
Like ET

I love you, I say
Yes, he says because how could I not
Yes, of course I do, how could it be otherwise

I make up foolish songs in operatic style
He chortles and squirms in embarrassed delight
To be silly is to feel safe, to be able to breathe

He tidies his room and eats his sandwich
And I watch
Rituals of the quotidian
Amongst so much change, so many little deaths
We find new norms, new patterns
Until it's time to say goodbye
No hug, no touch, just glass

Do you want the penguin I ask, we like penguins
They make us laugh
Curious little men in their formal attire
Tapping their feet to their inner rhythm
Yes, he says. I stand, move away, prepare to penguin
He is looking into the camera now
Watching, waiting as I stand, move towards him
Arms stiff to the side, waddle, waddle, flap, flap, hug
And, he grins, his melon slice smile, secure
In the knowledge that I am barmy and he is loved
Finger to finger we press the phone, white on red
Frozen for a second, then gone
My heartsong

MISSING

It is four hours since he went missing
It is dark now and Halloween
A night that amplifies my fears and inner screams
He does not see the edges of things
Cannot judge the speed of cars
Always is with others
Not a solo voyager, no intrepid adventurer he
The world makes him anxious, confuses and perplexes
Tonight it is Halloween
And it is four hours since he went missing
They think
For they are not sure exactly when he absconded
He took his bus pass but no phone
People are out looking
Police are informed
Bus and train stations, description given
I am asked where he might go
Perhaps to where he was meant to be
But was unable to be taken
He felt let down, disgruntled and betrayed
But he does not know the way
So follow the bus route he knows
And might have taken
It is over four hours since he went missing
It is dark and Halloween
I have aged ten years and vomit up my fears, again

Search the places where he feels safe
The places that are familiar
He has not been seen
Tonight is Halloween
There is far too much to look at
He will pass by unnoticed

My eyes and brain play tricks
Play me scenes I do not wish to see
He is so vulnerable, how could they let him go
I bargain with gods I do not altogether believe in
Keep him safe, please just keep him safe
It is dark, it is Halloween and now many hours
Since he went missing

My phone rings, it is where he used to live
He is at their door cold, scared and weeping
They give him shelter, keep him safe
Reassure him that no one is angry, just relieved
He wants to hear my voice
And so I speak gently to the sound of his sobs
Where he lives now, have been informed
Are on their way to take him home

Some days later he wants, with me
To retrace all the steps he has taken
On what we now call his adventure
And we do
Every bus stop, zebra, pelican too
Every junction, pavement, alleyway
The superstore, the marina, the waterside decking
I learn every pathway that he has taken
And thank the gods that watched over him
And brought him back albeit shaken
Though
Proud too of all those steps that he had taken

MAGIC NUMBERS

So, he says, I've got the dates
I have them written down, he says
He holds the pages to the screen
I see the dates writ large and clear
Two dates that speak such volumes
A date in May, a date in June
Magic numbers filled with promise
Numbers Seventeen and Twenty One

His hopes, his dreams stuck like glue
To these his magic numbers
He has been told
Heard and seen it on the news
Watched each and every briefing
It is writ large for him to see
Believes it must be going to be
It will, it has to happen

He has been robbed, he is deprived
Of people, things we know and trust
Of hugs, dancing and shouts of glee
Of the air upon his face
Hands are washed, gel applied
Mask is worn, glasses steam
Isolation
Meals forsworn, gigs abandoned

Holidays no more
He keeps the rules because we must
Get out of this pandemic
I am in awe
Of new found skills
That keep us still entangled

Covid will be ending on June 21st, he says
A magician waving his wand
We will be back to normal, he says
Things might not be just as they were, say I
Things might not be completely normal, say I
We might still need to wear a mask
And to keep a distance
We have been promised
We have been told
And we will not need to wear a mask
It really will be ending, he says
Covid is finished on June the twenty first

It is not easy to be in lockdown, he says
I do not feel so good
I broke a window, he says
My feelings are too big
I do not know where to put them
To talk is good, say I
It is he says don't go away
I stay

WHAT IF

Did you know
Did I know what
You know before he was born
Did you have a test
A test for what, I ask
Why make it easy for this total stranger
Who stands before us
Blocking our pushchair way
Her crass presumption
Her sense of entitlement
Worn like a garment, along with her lipstick
A test for what, I ask again
My thoughts drift, slip away
Did they know before you were born
That you would be crass and insensitive
Could the world have been spared
Your blundering foulness
The intrusive judgements of your kin
Relatives polarised and divided
Those who sought to reassure that
God loves all that he creates
So, he will have god's love just not theirs
Then those who grieved he would never be
The dentist, doctor, accountant or lawyer
And brought us smoked salmon and chopped liver

What if I had known
When I was told he might not walk or talk or feed unaided
What if I had known then
He would ask for scallops and linguine
When a visitor to tea
What if I had known then
That I would stand in a hardware store
Thinking fabulous fricative and
Hiccoughing to say
It's a bucket darling, b,b, bucket
It's a blue bucket
Whilst all stared at the potty mouthed child

What if I had known then
That I would lose him in the supermarket
And locate him sitting in the chilled cabinet
Smeared from head to toe
Eating a strawberry mousse

What if I had known then
We would one day go shopping
With no trail of destruction behind us
Shelves would remain stacked
Pyramids of cans intact
And toilet rolls unravelled not

What if I had known
We would stand at the checkout
And he would say loud and clear
Mummy Mummy Mummy
He was going through a phase of three being better than one
Yes I say
Mummy Mummy Mummy
Yes I say again
Putting items on the conveyor belt
Mummy Mummy Mummy
Yes sweetypops, what is it
Did you know, breath, did you know, bigger breath
Know what darling
By this time
He has not just my attention
The entire store is transfixed, frozen in time
Eyes are upon him, on us, agog
What is this thing I do not know
What is this breaking news
Did you know – pause long pause I – I
I have really hairy nuts
Do you darling, how lovely
My voice rising by at least three octaves
Wiping away tears of laughter
Hoping this particular news
Will not be shared publicly again

Information given he continues packing the bags

Oh yes, what if I had known all this then
She is still there, her lips are moving
You know a test to see, so you could choose
I wonder, I say to
She who will not budge
I wonder, given a choice
Would your mother have chosen you

Meanwhile he smiles up at me
And hands me his sock
A gift